Home Gym Handbook

6 Simple Steps To Start Working Out & Losing Weight TODAY!

Meghan Goode

Absolute Author
Publishing House

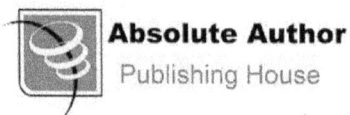

Home Gym Handbook
Copyright © 2023 Meghan Goode
Ms. Fitness Depot LLC

Publisher: Absolute Author Publishing House

Papberback ISBN: 978-1-64953-772-0
eBook ISBN: 978-1-64953-773-

TABLE OF CONTENTS

Important Note:

The information contained in this guide is not intended to be a substitute for professional medical advice, diagnosis or treatment. Do not self-diagnose or self-treat. Always seek the advice of your physician or other qualified health provider with any questions you may have regarding your condition. Never disregard professional medical advice or delay in seeking it because of something you have read in this guide.

GOALS ARE UNREACHABLE WITHOUT COMMITMENT

ABOUT THE AUTHOR

Meghan Goode is a fitness industry guru and healthy lifestyle advocate who went through a personal transformation and discovered how much of a struggle it was to get started on her fitness journey alone. As a result, she wrote Home Gym Handbook to provide a resource to serve as a starting point for women who are desperate for change, ready to start working out and living a healthy lifestyle, but are not quite sure where or how to start. This short book will offer the support you need to get started and stay on track. If you are ready to become a better version of yourself, then this is the book for you!.

COMMITMENT

If you've bought this book, then you've taken the first step of becoming a better YOU! However, before we move forward, I need you to commit to taking action to become your best self. Just buying the book isn't enough. You have to be willing to commit to taking the steps necessary to improve your life and most importantly your health. To help hold yourself accountable, I want you to write down this statement in your journal then sign and date it.

"Starting today, I will use 'The Home Gym Handbook' to take action steps in order to become my best self. I know that just reading the book is not enough. I know that I must follow the steps and put them into action in order to improve my life and health."

Sign:

Date:

Writing this statement in your journal will help you hold yourself accountable. Be sure to come back and read it often so you can remember what you promised yourself. Making changes to get better can get tough, but you are making this commitment to yourself.

Not only do I want you to make this commitment to yourself, I also want you to make a bold statement about what you want to do. Write out exactly what you want to achieve by the time you finish this book. Be specific in what you want and put it in writing. Here's an example:

"I, Meghan Goode, am making a commitment today to take action in becoming my best self. I commit to becoming healthier in the way I eat and becoming healthier physically. I understand that to achieve these goals, I have to set my goals and take action towards accomplishing them, no matter how difficult it may seem. I vow to push through the hard times because I know at the end of my journey I am going to become a better and happier ME!"

Signed,
Meghan Goode

REMEMBER WHY YOU STARTED

INTRODUCTION

How many times have you promised yourself that you were going to lose weight and get back into shape? How many times have you started a new program only to give up after a week or two because it just wasn't working for you? Enough is enough! There's no point in starting something if it's going to be a hassle. The many benefits of diet and exercise are obvious but making the decision to start can sometimes be the hardest part.

When you make the decision to hire a personal trainer, join a gym, start a fitness journey, or make better food choices, it can be a little overwhelming. It's hard to figure out where to start. How do you know whether or not this is something that will work for you?

It's okay to be nervous when taking such a big and important step. Before you do though, you're going to want to have a good idea of what you can expect. What is an ideal healthy weight for me? How much will I need to exercise? What foods will I be able to eat? How will I make time to exercise? Will I have to spend more money at the grocery store? There are so many questions!

It's not easy to ask someone else to help you change for the better. After all, as humans, we're all creatures of habit. It's true. When you wake up in the morning and brush your teeth, you do it the same way every time. You drive to work on the same route, even if there's a much shorter one available. And when you go to lunch with your friends, you always order the same thing.

These daily routines are good—they help us feel comfortable, safe and secure. But sometimes, it's important to step back and take a closer look at those habits, acknowledging the fact that they aren't always as good as they could be, and maybe you have some very unhealthy habits. Sometimes we need to change how we do things because doing what we've always done isn't working anymore.

This book is not only for those of you who need to lose weight and get in better shape now, but it is also for the people out there who are looking for a way to commit to self-improvement, better fitness and nutritional habits they can live with for the long term.

Do you want to get in shape, lose weight and gain muscle? Are you looking for motivation and support in your journey?

If you answered yes to any of these questions, then this book is for you!

FITNESS MINDSET

Motivational speaker Tony Robbins says, 'If you want to get off the island, you have to burn the boats.' This means get rid of all excuses and GO ALL IN. You have to figure out how you will reach your goal regardless of the obstacles which you might encounter along the way. There are no other options.

Most people skip over the subject of mindset, but I am a believer it is the gateway to any success in life. I believe that you must first change your mindset and believe you are more than capable of achieving any goal which you set your mind and intentions to attain. You are the only one who knows what you're willing and capable of doing.

As we jump into the meat and potatoes of the book, it's imperative for you to start with the right mindset. Finding what motivates you, finding a way to be held accountable, and getting over the initial fear of starting are the first steps to creating the best version of you. You will no longer make excuses to not live your best life.

Keep the bar high and raise your standards from what you have currently allowed up to this point. Keeping yourself accountable is the only option. You have to keep pushing and remember your only competition is staring back at you in the mirror. Your daily actions will decide if you are willing to do whatever it takes to reach your goals.

Don't Make Excuses
Make Results!

YOU DON'T
HAVE TO
BE GREAT TO
GET
STARTED, BUT
YOU
HAVE TO GET
STARTED
TO BE GREAT!
-ZIG ZIGLAR

CHAPTER 1: GETTING STARTED

So you are ready to start working out and you're ready to bring sexy back, huh?!

How hard can it be to get back into the swing of working out or to even start working out, I hear you ask! "I'm an ex-high school or college athlete and I know what it takes to get back in shape." This is what we tell ourselves. I walked past the bathroom mirror and had to do a double take because I didn't recognize the person staring back at me. I mean….of course we notice when we put on a few extra lbs from COVID and the pandemic but it's not THAT BAD! This is what we've been telling ourselves for weeks or even months now and finally this is the last straw. I decided to clean out our fridge and get rid of all the junk food, ice cream, and frozen dinners and everyone in the house was going on a diet whether they wanted to or not. Starting first thing Monday morning, I'm going to start working out again and eating healthy. I'm fired up and excited!!

Monday morning rolls around and the alarm goes off, but I hit snooze 5 times and now it's time to get ready for work or time to get the kids ready for school. So I decided to start tomorrow morning. Then I remembered that I have a doctor's appointment first thing in the morning, so I will have to postpone the workout until Wednesday morning. Since I threw away all of the groceries, I have to order takeout for dinner for the next couple of nights because I don't feel like going to the store after work or after picking up the kids from daycare. Does this sound familiar?

Now, you're probably reading this and thinking, 'Meg, that's where I am currently.' Trust me I totally understand. We must change the way we view health, wellness, and fitness and adopt a new mindset and way of thinking.

Adding a new workout plan into my busy life right now is not at the top of my list especially with how busy and hectic my schedule is, so I lose my motivation for getting back into shape.

Then one day while coming out of the bank I run into an old classmate from high school and I look like a hot mess and she is looking fly! I just want to crawl under a rock and hide and as we are saying our goodbyes she mentions telling people on FB that she ran into me. At that moment, my life flashes before my eyes and I say…..what has happened to me? Who have I become? How did I end up in this horrible place and lose myself and my 'SWAG'?!

The final straw was waking up one morning and feeling somewhat bloated. I proceeded to start my day like normal by heading to the bathroom to turn on the shower so the water could start to get hot. As I turned around, I glanced in the mirror and had to do a double take because I did not recognize the stranger looking back at me!!

OMG…..around my abdomen area I was bloated and appeared to be 3, maybe 4 months pregnant! My fingers looked like miniature sausage links, my face looked like I had jaw breaker candy in each cheek and my eyes were puffy as if someone had kicked my butt in my sleep (especially since I didn't have on my fake eyelashes first thing in the morning)! Enough is enough. What was really holding me back from starting the journey to feeling better about myself? The anxiety and the unknown which lay ahead was getting the best of me.

Showing up to the gym and not knowing anyone or deciding to start working out alone was not giving me the euphoric feeling which I had imagined. I'm guessing there are others who can relate and have experienced this state of being lost and in an unfamiliar place which can be scary, especially if you don't know how to fix it.

Can you totally relate? Maybe you are having the same feelings. You feel overweight, out of shape, low energy, bloated, and unattractive….. So, how do you get from where you are now back to your old self? How can I help you get from overweight and depressed to shedding pounds and living your best life in the shortest amount of time? Keep reading, because I'm going to show you how to be the best version of YOU!

I am going to provide you with some tips to help you become your best self. When you're done reading this book, you will have the motivation needed to become your best self, which is what you've been missing.

Your Next Steps Are To:

1. Admit you have not been taking care of yourself.

2. Write down what you want to change or what you want to do better in your life.

3. Commit to making a change.

A year from now, you will wish you started today!

IS IT 'ONE DAY' OR "DAY 1?"

CHAPTER 2: SETTING YOUR GOALS

I want to stop for a second and pass along one of my dirty little secrets. For years, one of my affirmations has been to get back in the best shape of my life in order to start officiating college basketball again.

After you've made the decision to start becoming a better YOU, you have to set goals. A goal is something you want to achieve. It is measurable whether it is how much money you want to earn, how much weight you want to lose, what size pants you want to fit into, etc. Without goals, it's impossible to know what you are working toward. If you don't have an end to reach, it will be impossible to stay on track and work toward what you want. It's hard to be successful and hold yourself accountable if you don't set goals that tell you what you want to accomplish. Here's how you can get started on goal setting:

- Make a list of some things you would like to accomplish. It could be food related, exercise related, etc.
- Be specific about the goals. Don't just say "I want to lose weight." Say how much weight you want to lose and by what date.
- Make an action plan of what steps you need to take to reach each goal. Be very detailed in what you need to do.
- Write down the things that have stopped you from achieving your goals before.
- Write out an action plan on how you are going to keep these things from stopping you this time. That way if one of those roadblocks comes up, you already have a plan in place.
- Make a commitment. Write out a commitment statement stating what your goal is, when you are going to achieve it, and what steps you are going to take to accomplish your goal. Sign your statement and be sure to read it every day.

Ready to make a change? Now's the time!

Your Next Steps Are To:

1. Take your list of goals and be sure they are as specific as you can get them. Create an action plan for achieving these goals.

2. Plan ahead for roadblocks that can sabotage your goals.

3. Write out your commitment statement to hold yourself accountable.

Take action now and commit to holding yourself accountable.

IF YOU DO WHAT
IS EASY, YOUR
LIFE WILL BE
HARD.

IF YOU DO WHAT IS
HARD, YOUR LIFE
WILL BE EASY.

-LES BROWN

CHAPTER 3: ENVISION YOUR GOALS

Let's be real: you want to look good naked.

Trust me, I know how hard it is to stay motivated and focused on the long-term goal of getting hardcore ripped with six-pack abs which some people dream about. For others, it's just about losing a few pounds so you don't get winded walking up and down the stairs.

It's a good idea to take some time and write down what you want out of your health goals. You don't want to just state your goals; you want to truly see them manifesting right in front of you. I'm talking about setting yourself up for success by setting SMART fitness goals—Specific, Measurable, Attainable, Relevant, and Timely. Your first step is to figure out what your goals are. First ask yourself these questions to figure out your goals.

1. What is your 'WHY'?
2. How will it change your life?
3. Break it down into something you can measure.
4. Make a schedule with milestones so you can figure out how you're going to achieve it.

SMART Goals

Once you know what goals you want to achieve, write them out following the SMART structure. Use the questions below to create your goals.

S   Specific - What do I want to accomplish?

M   Measurable - How will I know when it is accomplished?

A   Achievable - How can the goal be accomplished?

R   Relevant - Does this seem worthwhile?

T   Time Bound - When can I accomplish this goal?

Now that you have your goals in writing, now what? Ever heard the phrase, "out of sight, out of mind"? Well, that's exactly what happens when you don't have a vision board. If you have a goal in mind, it has to be visualized in some way, otherwise it can be easy to forget about it entirely.

We are seeking change once and for all so jotting them down then stashing them away in a junk drawer is not an option!

This should become a daily habit which will become stored in your subconscious mind to remind yourself of the healthy new you that you are striving to be.

You need something tangible that will help keep your motivation strong! Being laser focused on exactly what you want and your plan for making it happen.

This brings me to step #2.......vision boards. Vision boards are all over the internet these days. Pinterest is full of them! They're for people who want to travel the world and see all its wonders. But they're also for people who want to get healthy and lose weight. That's right—you can use a vision board to help you achieve your health goals as well!

Many personal trainers tell their clients that one thing that helps them most is visualization. The more vivid your mental picture of your goal is, the easier it will be for you to remember what it is and how you'll get there.

So take all those written goals that you have—the ones on paper or in your head—and bring them to life through visual aids like vision boards.

By doing this, you can keep yourself motivated without having to rely on willpower alone—and if you do forget about it for a while (hey! We're only human), then just pull out your vision board again!

Here are some tips for creating a vision board:

1. Take note of what inspires you in your life—whether it be a quote from someone important or a picture from Pinterest—and post it on your vision board to remind yourself why you want this goal in the first place.

2. Make sure each item on your board and your quote has meaning behind it and represents something that matters to you personally. Stick with only 5-7 items on your board at any given time; otherwise it can get overwhelming!

For example, if your goal is to lose 10 pounds in three months, take a picture of yourself at your current weight and put it on the board with an image of how much lighter you want to be by that time frame.

You can also put up images of what you will look like after those three months are up—maybe these are pictures of your favorite outfit on someone who has already reached this goal?

Another idea is to take pictures of foods that help you stay on track with your diet plan—this could include photos of healthy snacks like fruit or veggies (a few different kinds), or maybe even some kind of treat from time-to-time when you really deserve it!

3. Create an inspirational quote for yourself and write it down on sticky notes so they can be easily moved around. The key is not to let yourself get overwhelmed by having too many things on your list at once; focus on one thing at a time and take it from there!

4. You don't have to be a "vision board" expert to get the most out of this tool. The process is simple: choose images that represent what you want in life (like happiness and success), cut them out and glue them onto a poster board or cork board. Make sure they're big enough so that you can see them from across the room—you want these images to stand out and motivate you!

5. You can even create a digital vision board using Canva and create a wallpaper for your phone instead.

Your Next Steps Are To:

1. Create goals that follow the SMART structure.

2. Create a vision board of your goals.

3. Keep your vision board where you can see it daily. If it is digital, consider making it the wallpaper on your phone or on your computer.

BONUS OFFER

To help you get started, I have included a FREE Digital Vision Board which you can create in Canva.

Scan the QR Code below and make a copy of the board in Canva! Then get started on creating your digital vision board and bring your goals to life.

ACT LIKE THE PERSON YOU WANT TO BECOME

CHAPTER 4: WHAT IS YOUR MAIN GOAL?

Health goal specifics vary from person to person, but in general, the main goal whether weight loss, weight gain, or better eating habits, it is always to become a healthier version of you!

You may want to lose 5 pounds because you want to feel more confident in your body. You may want to gain 10 pounds because you want to build muscle and be stronger. Or maybe you just want to eat better because it makes you feel good about yourself and what you're putting into your body. Whatever the case may be, there are many ways that someone can become healthier.

The best way to start on this journey is by creating an action plan with small goals that are easy for you to achieve at first so that you will continue moving forward towards your final goal without feeling overwhelmed or discouraged along the way. When it comes to your goals, it's important to make sure you're setting yourself up for success. When you're deciding on your goals, ask yourself the following questions:

1. What is my ideal weight? Schedule an appointment with your physician and discuss with them what your personal, ideal Body Mass Index and Weight should be. While you can easily search the internet to find out what your weight should be, your healthcare professional can look at your medical history and take everything into consideration before giving you a number. This is especially important if you're on medication that slows down your metabolism. Once you have that number, write it into your Vision Board.
2. What are my fitness goals? Is it to lose weight? Gain strength? Tone up?
3. What do I want my body to look like? Write down how much fat or muscle mass you want to gain or lose, as well as any other physical characteristics (such as muscle tone). You may also want to include how often you plan on exercising and eating healthy foods in this section as well!
4. What areas of your body do you feel need the most work? If you want slender arms and legs, then print out stock images of your ideal look and post them on your Vision Board. The same goes for any other body part that you want to change. It's also a good idea to post pictures of exercises designed to tone those areas! Remember, be realistic with your expectations and base them on your body, not the model in the picture.

Write down all of your answers along with a time frame for achieving this goal (i.e., "Lose 20 pounds by December 31st"). You'll be amazed at how much easier it is to achieve your goals once you have a visual reminder of what they are.

The key is not to let yourself get overwhelmed by having too many things on your list at once. Focus on one thing at a time and take it from there!

Your Next Steps Are To:

1. Find out your ideal weight for your Age & Height.

2. Create achievable goals that target physical characteristics, like muscle tone or stronger core stability.

3. Finally set yourself up with small wins along the way so success is in sight.

Write down a time frame for achieving these goals and make sure they are SMART goals.

ARE YOU GOING THROUGH IT OR GROWING THROUGH IT?

CHAPTER 5: ROME WASN'T BUILT IN A DAY

When you decide to change your life, it's an exciting time. You're making a commitment to yourself, and that's the first step to creating a better future for yourself.

But sometimes, when we make big changes like this, we can get a little overwhelmed by all of the things we need to do. And when our brain senses this feeling of overwhelm, it starts to panic and tries to derail us from making those changes.

Don't let it! Instead, try slowing down the process just a bit as you make these decisions. Change is scary no matter what it is—whether it's changing your diet or creating a new career path—and your brain will use any excuse it can find to keep you from taking those steps forward. But if you take the time to slow down and really think about what you want out of life, then your brain will be able to accept these changes without trying so hard to fight them off.

When you're starting out, you don't have to do a lot to get results. You don't have to run a marathon every day, or even every week.

You don't even have to hit the gym five times a week.

You just need to start somewhere—and that somewhere can be as small as replacing one meal a day with something healthier, or doing a five-minute cardio session before your first cup of coffee in the morning.

The first step to a healthy lifestyle is making small changes that you can stick with, and you'll be amazed at how easy it is to build on these changes and make them stick.

Try one of these options and see where it takes you!

1. Instead of eating out every day, try having one meal at home each day. You might start with oatmeal and a piece of fruit—and then add in some protein on the side. That way you can still enjoy your coffee while getting some extra nutrients into your body.
2. If you're new to exercising, start by doing five minutes of cardio every morning before work or school—you can even do it while watching TV! Once you're ready for more intense workouts, schedule them with a personal trainer who will help guide you through proper technique.
3. You've probably heard this hundreds of times, but getting enough water really is one of the most important things you can do for yourself every day.

It's not an easy switch from soda, though. Start out slow by replacing an eight-ounce cup of water for one serving of soda per day. From there, move up as quickly as you can, until water is your main source of hydration.

It can be tempting to get a little extra flavor in your H20, but try to keep it simple at first and stick with just plain water. When you start craving more, try using lemon slices or cucumber slices to add some flavor without the calories (and sugar).

Don't forget about other drinks that count toward your daily water intake! Coffee, tea, and milk are all included in the total amount of fluid you should consume each day—so don't feel like you need to drink more just because you love coffee!

Your Next Steps Are To:

1. Commit to swapping unhealthy snacks with something healthier.

2. Increase your activity level by increasing your cardio each week.

3. Don't forget that staying hydrated is key for fueling yourself properly - grab an extra glass or two throughout the day.

Take the first step today and you'll be surprised by what can come of it!

PROGRESS

NOT

PERFECTION

CHAPTER 6: REPLACE OLD HABITS

This time of year is all about self-reflection and planning for the future. If you want to make 2023 your best year yet, it's important to take a look at how you can make some changes in your life.

If you want to lose weight or tone up, it's going to take more than a couple of weeks. Unfortunately for most of us, old habits die hard. This is why we are going to select a slow and steady pace from the beginning. With just a few small changes to your old habits, you can begin to eat healthier and you can add in that short 10 minute cardio session in the morning to get you going and start your day off with a win.

The best way to start is by doing something that's easy to stick with, so you can build up momentum and get comfortable with the routine. That way, we can build up your strength and endurance gradually over time—instead of trying to do too much at once and getting discouraged right away.

<u>Here are a few tips on how to change those habits:</u>

1. Grocery Shopping

We've all been there: you're grocery shopping and you just want to get in and get out. You don't have time for anything fancy, and you definitely don't want to be standing in line forever.

You're looking for the fastest way to do your shopping, and we know how you feel—we've all been there! You go through the motions, throwing cartons of ice cream and bags of chips in the cart without question. But is it really helping?

If you've found yourself doing this without thinking, it's time to regroup. We know it can seem like a lot of effort at first, but if you're serious about making your grocery shopping routine more efficient and effective, then we have some tips for you!

Let's start with the basics: grab a list! That's right—a list! Having a list keeps you focused on what items are most important to purchase at the store, instead of running around aimlessly trying to remember them all. It also makes sure that nothing slips through the cracks when it comes time to check out—no more forgetting things like toilet paper or toothpaste at home!

Cooking is hard. And eating healthy is even harder. So let us help you make it easier.

Here's the deal: if you want to eat healthy and make a difference in your life, it's not enough to just make a few changes here and there—you have to make systemic changes that will stick with you for years to come.

The good news is that we've got the perfect solution for you! All you need to do is swap out one food each week when you shop and then build on that.

So what does this mean? Let's say you buy nothing but frozen pizzas and ice cream. You could swap out your regular carton of ice cream for a low-fat version of your favorite flavor! Or maybe instead of buying chicken nuggets, try out some chicken breasts or thighs! The possibilities are endless!

Once you start swapping one bad food with one healthy one each week when you shop, it won't be long before your body starts craving junk food less often than ever before!

2.   Set Your Clothes Out the Night Before

It's so easy to get up in the morning and realize that you've forgotten something. But if you remember to set your clothes out the night before, you'll be more likely to have everything ready to go!

This will save you time in the morning and leave you feeling less rushed and frustrated by giving you that extra time you need in the morning to do your short workout.

3.   Setup Your Coffee Maker

You might think this one is obvious, but we promise it works! It's amazing how much time it takes to set up a coffee maker—it's definitely worth doing before bed so you can wake up with a fresh pot of coffee ready for you each morning!

4.   Pack Your Lunch for Tomorrow

This one also seems like a no-brainer, but what happens when we forget? By packing your lunch ahead of time, not only will it save you time tomorrow morning (and make sure that nobody steals anything!), but it will also help keep things organized throughout the week! This will also allow you time to pack something healthy rather than being rushed at the last minute in the morning and just throwing whatever is convenient in your lunch bag.

Keep going and reap all those amazing benefits from making these small changes one at a time.

Your Next Steps Are To:

1. Don't let bad habits control your life! Create a grocery list that swaps out old, unhealthy items for healthier alternatives.

2. Take the time to lay out an outfit and have coffee ready each morning - these little steps can jump-start success in more areas of life than you think.

3. Save yourself some stress by preparing meals ahead of time; it'll take no effort when lunchtime comes around tomorrow!

Small changes will produce big results!

CONCLUSION

Congratulations are in order for finishing the book and investing in yourself by completing this book! I am so proud and confident in each of these 6 fitness strategies that you now have access to. Each one helped me kickstart my recent fitness journey, which means they will hopefully work for you as well with just some minor execution from your side. And here's what makes it all even better... if applied correctly, each tip could bring expedited results and weight loss success!

The road to fitness is not always easy, but it's worth the journey. If you're ready to make real sacrifices and push yourself beyond your limits, then this guide is for you.

To get in the best shape of your life, there will be real sacrifices that you will have to make. You'll need to be consistent about fitness and make it a real priority. You will also have to take the time to make sure that you are adequately celebrating your wins while holding yourself accountable.

You might also have to remain conscious about your relationships. It can be very challenging to get fit if you have a close friend or significant other who tries to tempt you into unhealthy activities, or has anything negative to say about your journey.

It's up to you to make sure that you let people know you are serious about your fitness journey. No matter what challenges come up along the way, you need to be consistent about fitness. It has to become a real priority for you. You have to take time out of each day to make sure that you are getting enough exercise and eating properly.

You'll also need to celebrate your wins, and hold yourself accountable when you slip up. Ultimately, it might not be easy—it may even be painful—but know that these sacrifices will pay off in the end: a body and mind that are strong, healthy, and ready for anything! In the end, your body and mind will thank you for getting fit!

Let's make an agreement right now – commit to using at least two methods starting today, then watch how much more successful life can be in a short period of time when used strategically together.

Now that you've taken the first step to unlocking your next level of success, I'm here to provide you with resources that can help you get where you want to be. Are you ready and serious about transforming and investing in yourself?

The ball is in your court, sis!!

There are also additional books and other resources which are available and more suited to your needs. To find out what will work best for you, scan the QR Code below and check out the other resources and GET STARTED TODAY!!

Thank You!

Thank you for taking the time to read my book. I know it can be a great resource in helping you reach your goals. Let's take action now! With every journey comes bumps in the road, but stay motivated and never stop striving towards progress. Reach out to me anytime if more guidance is needed, and get plugged into our community as taking these steps are crucial to success! Here's wishing nothing but much success on your journey!

Your friend and coach,

Coach Meg